What the Heck's for Breakfast?

Gluten and Grain Free Ideas to Reclaim Energy and Health
with the Most Important Meal of the Day

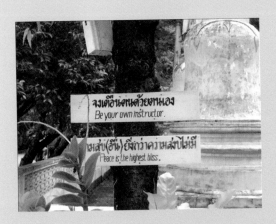

จงเตือนตนด้วยตนเอง
Be your own instructor.

...มสุข(อื่น)ยิ่งกว่าความสงบไม่มี
Peace is the highest bliss.

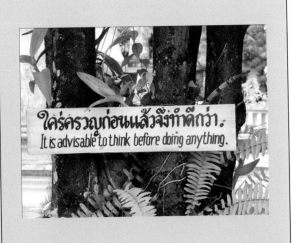

ใคร่ครวญก่อนแล้วจึงทำดีกว่า
It is advisable to think before doing anything.

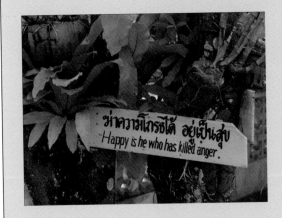

ฆ่าความโกรธได้ อยู่เป็นสุข
Happy is he who has killed anger.

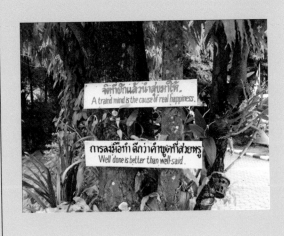

จิตที่ฝึกแล้วนำสุขมาให้
A traind mind is the cause of real happiness.

การลงมือทำ ดีกว่าคำพูดที่สวยหรู
Well done is better than well-said.

What the Heck's for Breakfast?
Gluten and Grain Free Ideas to Reclaim Energy and Health
with the Most Important Meal of the Day

By Tracy Roberge

Published by Tracy Roberge

2015

First Printing: 2015

ISBN 978-1-312-65708-3

Published by Tracy Roberge
tintinnabular@outlook.com
Calgary, Alberta, Canada

www.tintinnabular.com

 TT

Ordering information:

Special discounts are available on quantity purchases by corporations, associations, educators, and others. For details, contact the publisher at tintinnabular@outlook.com

Dedication

To my family and friends for always encouraging me.

To Jacob and Alec, who inspire me every day.
Thanks for putting up with all my crazy experiments in the kitchen.

All My Love

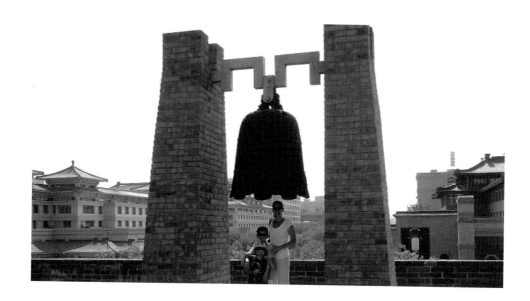

Contents

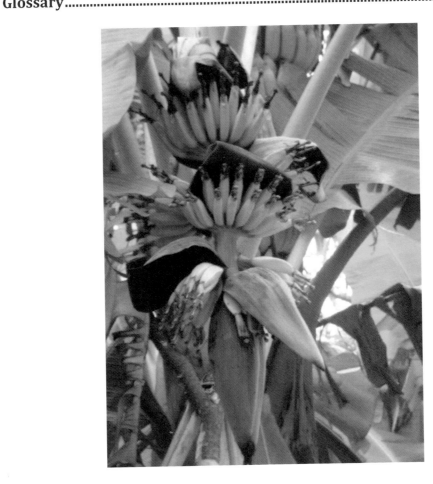

Introduction - Our Journey as a Family

When my son was an infant he broke out in a crazy rash all over his head. I took him to an allergist who prescribed zinc cream and we went on our merry way. When he was 3 years old, he started losing patches of hair. I was told it was either stress or a condition called alopecia (a form of hair loss). Again we went on our merry way. Then at the age of 5, my son began to experience severe cramps and sharp pains in his tummy. I was called from work several times a month to pick him up. The doctors told me he was just constipated and to give him more fiber. So I sprinkled oat bran in spaghetti sauce, high-fiber grains in cookies and yogurt, and served oatmeal whenever I could; after all, we are told grains are our best source of fiber. But the pain and constipation continued in my child, who also experienced a lack of focus and difficulty sleeping.

Finally, after one simple blood test, the results showed that my son wasn't processing gluten in the right range. Within weeks of putting him on a traditional gluten-free diet (meaning no wheat, barley, rye or oats) he made a significant improvement. The cramps dissipated, his sleep improved, his focus in school improved and he was a much happier child. As a parent you have to fight for your child when you know something is wrong. The same is true for yourself.

In 2010 my family moved from Calgary, Alberta in Canada (one of the world's cleanest places to live) to Hong Kong, China. Although I was quite often sick with colds, lack of energy and heartburn, within 6 months of moving I began experiencing a constant dull ache and throbbing in my right side. This progressed into a sharp piercing pain that kept me up all night, and ended in the morning with diarrhea the first few hours I was up. All tests came back normal. My celiac blood test was negative so I was still eating grains. Finally, after a colonoscopy I was diagnosed with IBS (Irritable Bowel Syndrome) and instructed to eat a "traditional" gluten-free diet (no wheat, barley, rye or oats).

The throbbing in my abdomen lessened, but I still had constant pain in my side and very difficult bowel movements every morning. Finally, in December 2012, my doctor referred me to a naturopath; a health-practitioner who favors a holistic approach to healing the body. I went through allergy testing and the results showed a reaction to all grains including traditionally safe ones like rice and corn – the staples on most gluten-free diets.

My digestive system was so compromised that I was reacting negatively to many other foods as well. What triggered this is still unclear; maybe it was exposure to so many new toxins in an unfamiliar country, or the stress of the move to the other side of the world. But what was very clear was that I could not eat grains.

The first couple of weeks were very stressful. Not only did I have to start a grain-free diet, I also had to avoid a number of foods that I had negative reactions to. I went through what felt like withdrawal from gluten and sugar, and had a really hard time figuring out what to eat because I had relied on rice flour and corn flour in most of my recipes. But after a few weeks I had more energy, and after a few months the throbbing in my side subsided.

I now depend on coconut flour and almond flour, and use honey, maple syrup or organic coconut palm sugar in my baking. These sweeteners are absorbed slowly into the bloodstream and unlike traditional cane sugar they do not cause a spike in the body's glycemic ratings.

My naturopath also tested the pH levels (acidity or alkalinity levels) in my body. It is recommended that the body be neutral at a reading of between 7.35 and 7.45. I tested on the acidic side, which can decrease the body's ability to absorb minerals and other nutrients. I was also put on vitamin D3, an omega supplement, a daily multi-vitamin and probiotics to help restore the healthy bacteria in my intestines and bring balance to my body. Once again, make sure any supplement you are on doesn't have gluten.

I won't get into specifics here, but it may be worth it for you to consult with a naturopath or homeopath for full testing. I truly believe every one of us is unique and different. We all have certain foods that our body needs and other foods we should avoid. Until you understand what foods you react to, you will be playing a guessing game and delaying your healing. Naturopaths or homeopaths can recommend vitamins and minerals where you may be deficient and this can help speed healing as well.

If you feel hesitant about considering alternative medicine or consulting a naturopath or homeopath, the advice I would offer is to look at the results traditional medicine has given you. A naturopath will provide you with options that you may not have with traditional medicine and can work in conjunction with your family doctor. A naturopath will open up the door to healing in a different way and create a holistic plan for you and your specific needs. Plus nowadays, many health insurance companies cover some consultation costs as they recognize the value that naturopaths offer.

After going on this journey of self-healing, I truly believe that the foods we put into our bodies help to heal and sustain us to live life to its fullest. So take charge of your healing. Find out what your body needs by visiting a naturopath to be allergy and PH tested and work with a holistic nutritionist once you know what your body needs. Most importantly, don't go hungry. Eat as much as you want, when you want, focusing on lots of fruits and vegetables. The best snack you can give yourself is a fruit, veggie or handful of nuts.

This book offers some basic but delicious recipes to support your own investigation into healthy eating. I developed these recipes and suggestions by trial and error after trying recipes from many sources. I discovered that most of them just didn't work out the way I wanted, or really needed modifications to taste half-decent. The recipes I am sharing with you are ones that have been given the thumbs up by my family. But you may find after trying them that you want to change a few things to your liking. Please do!

My final piece of advice is keep at it. There are so many resources at your disposal with the internet, blogs, and websites. Know that you are not alone.

To your health and getting that pizzazz back into your life!

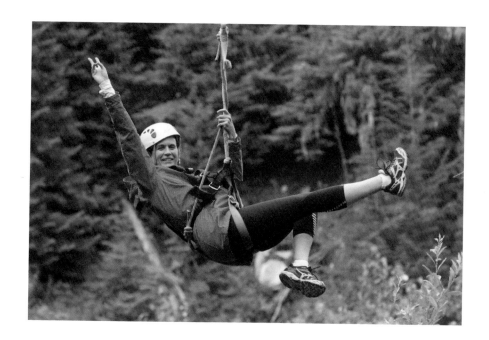

Eating Gluten/Grain-Free Tips

- Always check any bottled or packaged purchase for hidden wheat or various other grains (wheat, barley, rye, oats, corn, rice).
- Try to avoid anything thickened with corn starch. Corn is high in gluten so can affect your healing. It is commonly found in yogurt, sour cream, BBQ sauces and salad dressings.
- If a bottled item says "spices" it may contain wheat as a filler. Avoid it.
- If a bottled item says "other ingredients" it may contain gluten. Avoid it.
- Watch for corn starch or rice starch in your baking soda, and dairy products.
- My rule – if in doubt don't use it. You'll feel so much better!
- If it's fresh from the produce aisle, it's great! Hit this grocery aisle first.
- Do a search on line for Paleo recipes and start your own investigation.
- Coconut flour and almond flour are your new best friends for baking.
- Adopt smoothies for breakfast or an energy boost any time of the day.
- The best snack you can give your body is a fruit or veggie.
- Replace traditional cane sugar with organic coconut palm sugar. It has a glycemic rating of 35, meaning it's slowly absorbed into the bloodstream so it doesn't spike your blood sugars like regular sugar does. But don't go overboard. It's still a form of sugar.
- Don't dismiss a recipe if it has one or two ingredients you can't have. Find a way to be creative and replace or swap it out for another ingredient. Or try omitting it and see if it works.
- Always carry some dried fruits or nuts with you for when your blood sugars drop. This will help you avoid sugar crashes and the temptation to feed your body unwisely. Fuel your body with dried mango, figs, raisins, apricots, or any other unprocessed fruit without sugar. Nuts are also a great alternative, but make sure they are unsalted and unprocessed (avoid dry roasted).
- Try coconut water. It is loaded with magnesium and potassium, helping to replenish your electrolytes and rejuvenate you.
- Drink lots of water every day.

Breakfast Introduction

Breakfast was one of the most challenging meals of the day when my family first went gluten and grain-free. We were so used to grabbing that slice of toast or bagel; spreading a croissant with cream cheese or digging into that sugary bowl of cereal. Now the question was, what the heck were we going to have for breakfast?

The answer is actually quite simple. You can get sick of eggs every morning, but there are endless and wonderful alternatives with muffins, pancakes, or smoothies.

Truth be told, in the western world we eat way too many sugary carbs for breakfast anyway. And my family has found that the best breakfast by far-- and the simplest -- is the smoothie. At least 3-4 times a week this is our breakfast and it has so much more healthy fiber in it than a bowl of processed cereal or slice of toast.

But you be the judge. Enjoy some of these favorites from my kitchen to yours. And if something doesn't sit right with you, experiment with changing up the recipe to suit your needs or taste buds. So wake up with energy, and enjoy the first meal of the day!

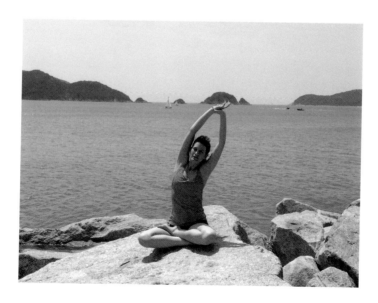

Apples and Nut Butter

This is so easy you'll wonder why I included it, but it's one of the easiest breakfast or snacks you can have.

There is a long list of health benefits attributed to apples due to the wealth of vitamins, minerals, nutrients, and organic compounds in them. Add the protein from peanut or cashew butter and this is so much better than toasting that processed bread for breakfast.

Prep time: 2 mins   *Serves: 1-2*

Directions:

Cut the apple into slices.

Scoop the nut butter onto a plate to dip, or directly onto the apple.

Voila! Instant, easy, nutritious breakfast.

Note: Peanuts are actually a legume, so if you are following a paleo diet, you may want to defer to the cashew or almond.

Ingredients:

➢ Apple
➢ Peanut, cashew or almond butter (use only natural butters with no oil or sugar added – but you can mix with in a bit of honey if you want it to taste sweeter)

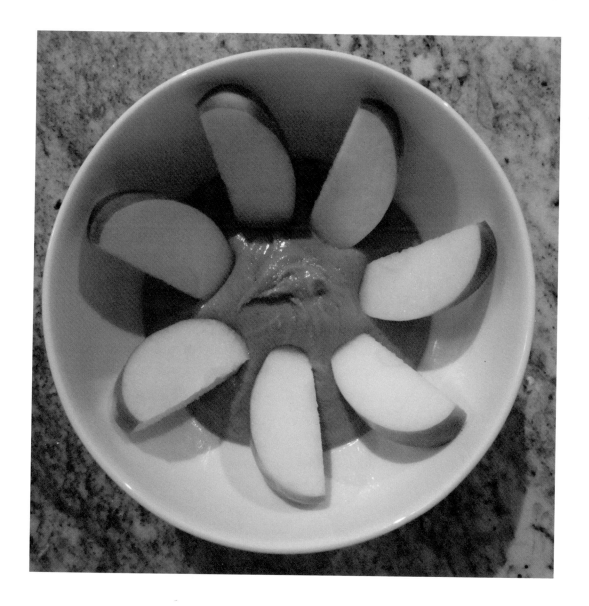

Avocado Baked Eggs

I love avocados, and this is a great recipe that provides a healthy serving of over 20 vitamins and minerals. Get ready for a big energy boost to start your day!

Your avocado may move around a bit in the pan so either balance it on the side of the sheet or trim the bottom to make it flat.

Prep time: 2 mins   *Serves: 1-2*

Directions:

Preheat oven to 425°F

Beat one egg with a fork.

Cut an avocado in half. Twist to open and remove the pit.

Place the avocado halves in a baking sheet, pitted side up, propped against the side to keep them steady.

Whisk egg in a bowl with salt and pepper to taste. Pour ½ the egg into the center of each avocado half. Place in the oven.

Bake for 15 minutes or until the egg is set.

Option:

Sprinkle spices or condiments on top. These are all good: chili powder, cumin, paprika or lemon zest.

Ingredients:

➢   1 avocado
➢   1 egg
➢   salt & pepper

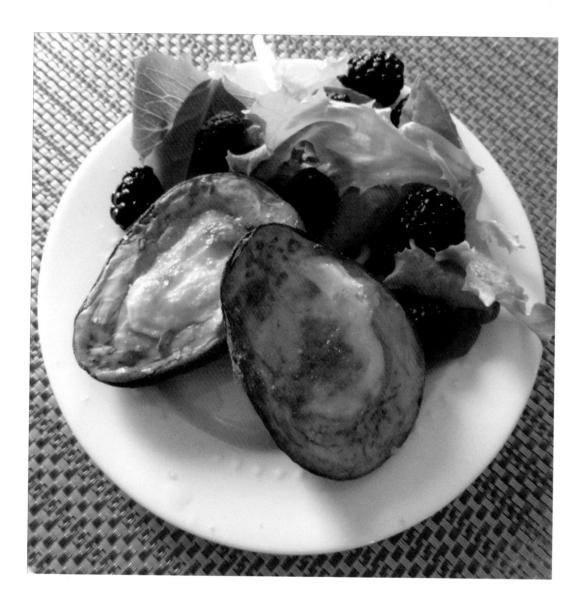

Banana Bread

Who says you can't go bananas over banana bread on a grain-free diet? This loaf will have you coming back for more.

My children love this recipe, and it's also nut free so they can also take it to school.

Prep time: 15 mins   *Serves: 8-12*

Directions:

Preheat oven to 350°F

Line 5x9 loaf pan with parchment paper and grease with coconut oil.

Remove pits from dates. Microwave dates with ¼ cup water for 30 seconds or until the dates have softened. Mash with a fork.

In a separate bowl, mash bananas and add to date mixture. Add eggs, vanilla extract, and honey and whisk together thoroughly.

In separate bowl, sift coconut flour, cinnamon, salt and baking soda.

Pour the liquid ingredients into the dry and mix well. Add melted coconut oil and mix well.

Mix in cacao nibs (or chocolate chips and any other options).

Spoon batter into prepared loaf pan.

Ingredients:

➢ 6 Mejool dates
➢ ¼ cup water
➢ 3 bananas
➢ 5 eggs
➢ ½ tsp vanilla extract
➢ ⅓ cup of honey
➢ ¼ tsp salt
➢ ¼ cup cacao nibs
➢ ½ tsp cinnamon
➢ ¾ tsp baking soda
➢ ½ cup sifted coconut flour
➢ ¼ cup coconut oil

Bake for 1 hour or until toothpick comes out clean. Remove loaf from the oven and let it cool for 5 minutes.

Run a knife along the edges and flip the loaf onto a flat surface or wire rack. Turn the loaf so the bottom is flat on the wire rack and let cool.

Option:

Add in ½ cup of raisins, walnuts or cacao nibs.

If you would like it to be sweeter, you can add in some chocolate chips when the batter is fully mixed. Just check the ingredients of the chips to make sure they are wheat free.

Optional:

➢ ½ cup walnuts, raisins, cacao nibs or chocolate chips.

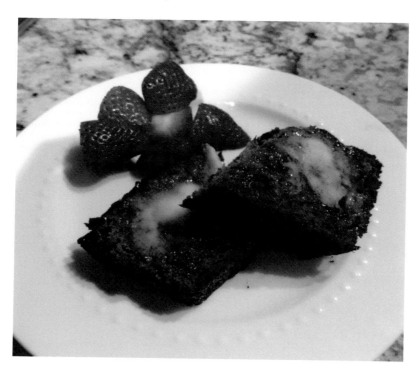

Blueberry Orange Mini Muffins

These mini-muffins are a hit, especially with cashew or almond butter on top for extra protein, or butter and jelly. They have a nice citrus flavor and are great nut free as well.

Wonderful to serve at a breakfast, tea or to take to school or the office. Pop one in your mouth and enjoy!

Prep time: 10 mins   *Makes: 24*

Directions:

Preheat oven to 350°F

Blend eggs, coconut oil/butter, vanilla, honey, orange juice and orange zest in a bowl.

Sift in the coconut flour, baking soda, and salt.

Fold in the blueberries.

Grease a mini-muffin pan.

Fill muffin pan ¾ full and bake for 25-30 mins, or until toothpick comes out clean.

Option:

You can do these as full size muffins as well, but increase baking time.

Ingredients:

➢ 6 eggs
➢ ½ cup coconut oil or butter
➢ 1 tbsp orange juice
➢ zest from 1 orange
➢ 1 tsp vanilla extract
➢ ¼ cup honey
➢ ½ cup coconut flour
➢ ½ tsp baking soda
➢ ½ tsp salt
➢ 1 cup fresh or frozen blueberries

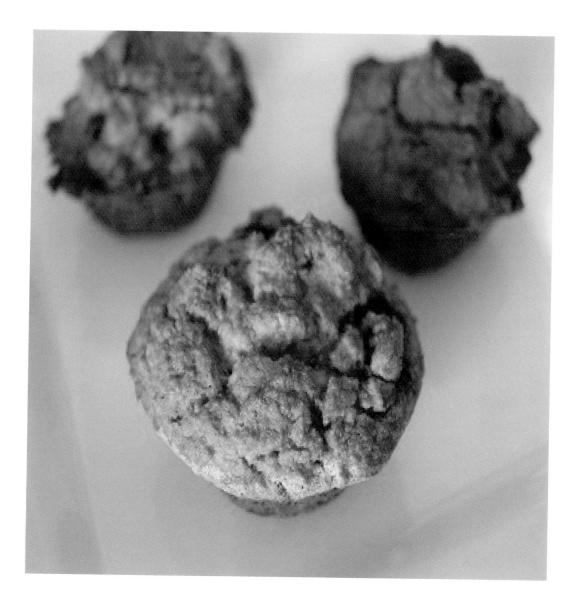

Banana Carrot Muffins

This recipe is so filling and yummy, and very hearty so it definitely will leave you feeling satisfied.

Protein from the nuts, vitamins and fiber from the carrots, banana and dates. It will be hard to stop at one.

Prep time: 15 mins   *Makes: 12*

Directions:

Preheat oven to 350°F

Grease muffin pan with coconut oil.

Heat dates with 2 tbsp water in microwave to soften. Mash with a fork and add mashed bananas to date mixture.

Add apple cider vinegar and melted coconut oil to banana/date mixture. Blend in the eggs.

Grind walnuts and pecans in food processor or blender. Add shredded carrots, cinnamon, sea salt and baking soda.

Add banana/date mixture to nut mixture and mix thoroughly.

Fill muffin pan ¾ full and bake for 25-30 mins, or until toothpick comes out clean.

Option:

Add in ½ cup raisins.

Ingredients:

- 3 eggs
- 3 bananas
- 1 cup pitted dates
- 1 tsp apple cider vinegar
- ½ cup melted coconut oil
- 1 ½ cups shredded carrots
- 1 tbsp cinnamon
- 1 tsp sea salt
- 2 tsp baking soda
- 2 cups walnuts
- ½ cup pecans

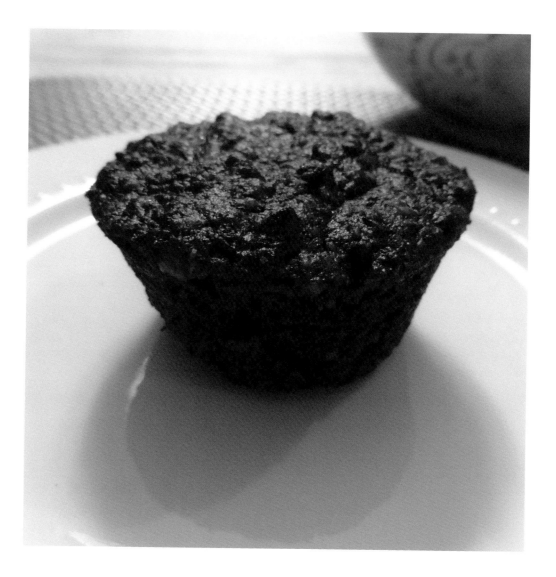

Bread

When first diagnosed I was also reacting to almonds and needed to avoid them. Most grain-free recipes called for almond flour, so experimenting with coconut flour became an obsession.

When the loaves are fully cooled, slice the bread into 1" thick slices and cover tightly with plastic wrap or freezer storage bags. Store in the freezer. Just pop a slice in the toaster when you need one.

Prep time: 10 mins   *Makes: 4 loaves*

Directions:

Heat oven to 350°F

Line the bottom of 4 small loaf pans (3"x6") with parchment paper and grease with coconut oil.

Mix all ingredients together in a large bowl, adding melted butter or coconut oil last.

Pour or scoop evenly into the 4 greased loaf pans.

Bake for about 35 minutes or until a toothpick inserted in the center of a loaf comes out clean.

Turn the baked bread onto a cooling rack and remove parchment paper from the bottom of each loaf. Turn loaves back over to cool fully.

Option:

If making a large loaf, add additional time (approx. 60 mins).

Ingredients:

- 12 eggs
- ¾ cup tapioca flour
- ¼ cup coconut flour
- 3 tsp apple cider vinegar
- 1 ½ tsp cream of tartar
- 1 ½ tsp baking soda
- ¾ cup melted butter or coconut oil

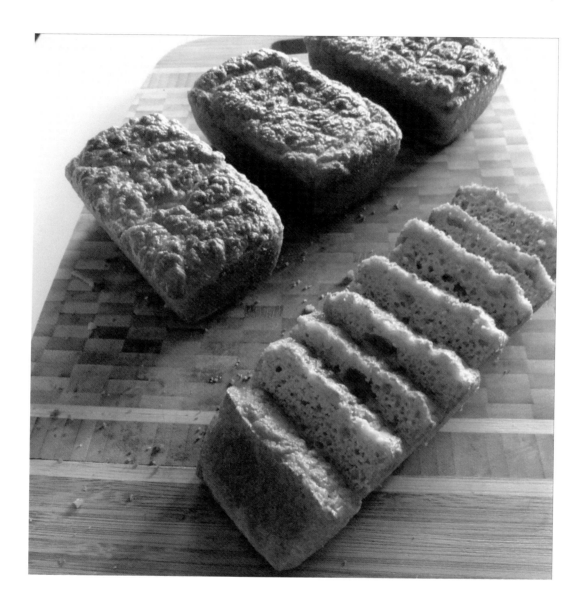

Cashew Butter Muffins

These are my most favorite muffin and are just delicious. They are so moist, but not mushy.

You can freeze them until you need them. Just cut them in half while they are still frozen and put them in the toaster oven for a warm breakfast treat.

Prep time: 10 mins   *Makes: 12*

Directions:

Preheat oven to 350°F

Grease a 12-muffin pan with coconut oil.

Mash bananas and add cashew butter to mix.

Stir in eggs and honey.

Add remaining ingredients, blending thoroughly.

If adding fruit, add last and mix in gently.

Scoop batter into muffin tin and bake for 15-20 mins, or until toothpick inserted in the center comes out clean.

Option:

Add ½ cup of fruit like blueberries, strawberries, raisins. For a special treat add ½ cup chocolate chips (look for brans without wheat, dairy or soy).

Ingredients:

➢ 1 cup organic cashew butter
➢ 2-3 mashed bananas
➢ 3 eggs
➢ ¼ cup honey
➢ 1 tsp vanilla extract
➢ 1 tsp baking soda
➢ 1 tsp cinnamon

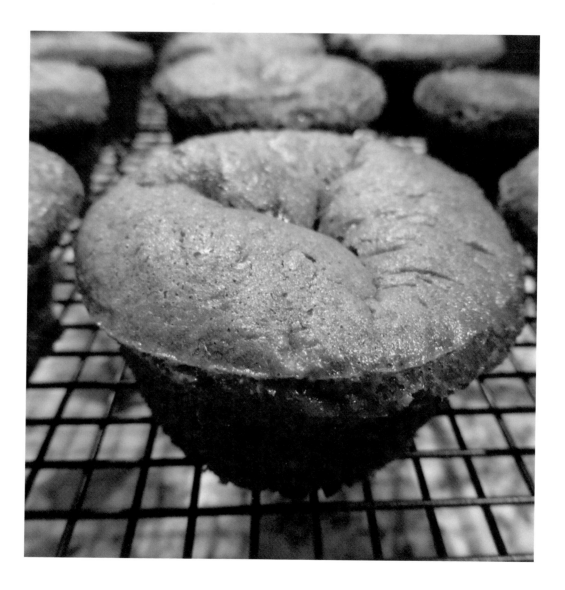

Cinnamon Rolls

Two words – Yum – my! The first time I made these my kids and I ate the entire batch within the day.

Most recipes I try tend to require a lot of massaging to make it just right. I had my doubts when I tried this one, but the results were fantastic. I just had to include it with full credit to a website called www.agirlworthsaving.net.

Prep time: 10 mins   *Makes: 12*

Directions:

Place the coconut oil, water and sea salt, maple syrup/honey in a small pan and bring to a boil. Let boil for 30 seconds.

Remove from the stove and add the tapioca flour in to the pan and mix with a spoon until you have a sticky dough.

Let this cool for 3- 4 minutes and then add in the coconut flour and egg.

Mix with a spoon until you have a soft dough and then remove from the pan and place on a piece of parchment paper. Knead for 1 minute.

Place a second piece of parchment paper over the top and then roll the dough into roughly a 7" x 11" rectangle that is ¼ thick.

For the filling combine the maple syrup/honey, cinnamon and water in a small bowl. Toss in the coconut flakes, nuts and raisins until well coated.

Ingredients Dough:

- ➤ ½ cup coconut oil
- ➤ ½ cup of water
- ➤ ½ tsp sea salt
- ➤ 1 cup tapioca flour
- ➤ ½ cup coconut flour
- ➤ 2 tbsp honey
- ➤ 1 large egg

Ingredients Filling:

- ➤ ½ cup unsweetened flaked coconut
- ➤ ½ cup chopped nuts
- ➤ ⅓ cup of raisins
- ➤ 1 tbsp honey
- ➤ 2 tbsp water
- ➤ ½ tsp cinnamon

Spoon this mixture evenly over the dough leaving a ½" board from the sides.

Now roll the dough into log and lightly press to pinch the seam.

Cut ¼" off the ends of and then slice into 1" pieces.

Place the slices and ends flat side down on to a piece of parchment paper and bake at 350 for 30 to 35 minutes.

For the frosting mix the palm shortening, coconut milk, maple syrup and cinnamon with a hand blender.

Remove the cinnamon rolls from the oven and let cool for 3 to 5 minutes. Frost with the frosting and enjoy!

Ingredients Frosting:

➤ ¼ cup palm shortening or butter
➤ 1 tbsp coconut milk
➤ 1 tbsp honey
➤ ½ tsp cinnamon

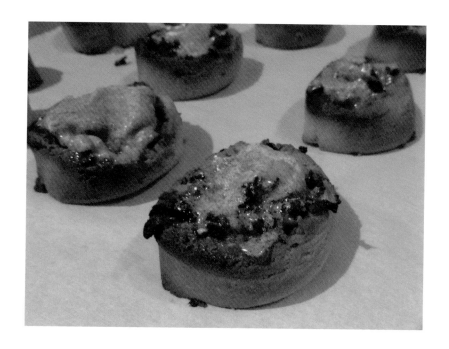

Date Nut Energy Balls

I discovered dates while living in Asia. I love their sweetness and how their pasty texture can be used for so many things.

This is a simple mixture of dates and optional add-ins that are guaranteed to satisfy your hunger and give you energy. And they're a great snack on the go as you're running out the door.

Prep time: 15 mins   *Makes: 12-15*

Directions:

Mash the pitted dates in a bowl. This is the binding agent that holds the mixture together.

In a chopper or food processor, pulse the nuts and salt until coarsely ground.

Add in any of your optional items.

You should be able to squeeze the mixture into a clump.

Roll the mixture into small bite-sized balls and store in refrigerator until ready to eat.

Optional Add Ins:

➤ 1/3 cup shredded coconut
➤ 1/3 cup chocolate chips or cacao nibs
➤ ½ cup raisins or your favorite dried fruit.

Ingredients:

➤ 2 cups pitted dates
➤ ½ cup pecans
➤ ½ cup cashews
➤ ½ cup sunflower seeds
➤ ¼ tsp salt

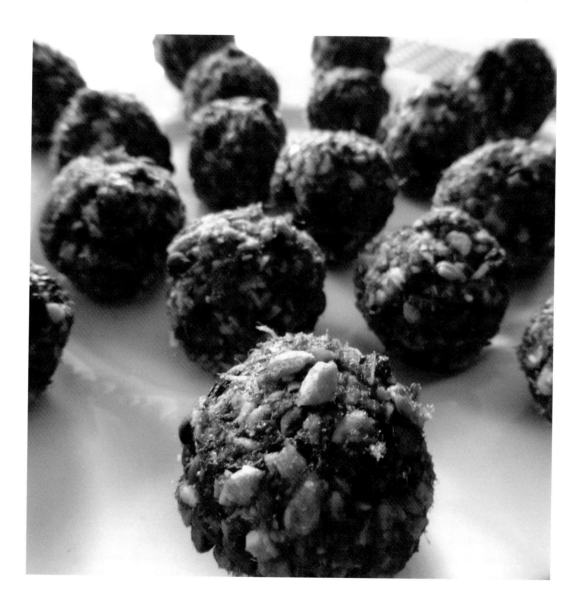

Egg Melt on Toast

My kids really enjoy this. It's full of fiber from the coconut in the bread and protein from the eggs.

Of course they also get a healthy serving of fruit on the side as well. It is a great way to start the day.

Prep time: 5 mins   *Serves: 1*

Directions:

Toast coconut bread.

While bread is toasting, break the egg in a heated frying pan, stirring gently to create a bit of a scramble before letting it settle.

Cook bacon separately, or use left-overs from a previous meal. I always keep a stash of cooked bacon in the fridge so I can put together this easy dish in a snap.

Once egg is cooked, place on toasted coconut bread.

Top with cheese and/or bacon. Put in toaster oven until cheese is melted. Can serve with a dollop of organic ketchup.

Optional:

Can also put sliced, nitrate free ham on top in place of the bacon.

Ingredients:

➢ Prepared bread (page 27)
➢ 1 egg
➢ Nitrate-free bacon (optional)
➢ 1 slice of cheese (optional)
➢ Organic ketchup (optional)

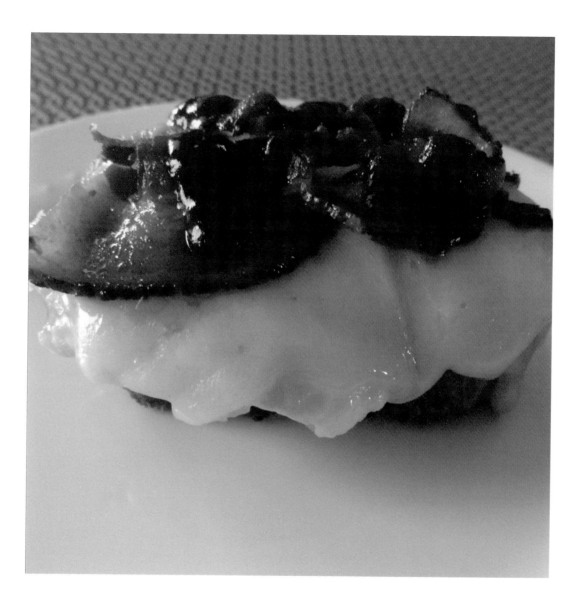

Granola Cereal

One of the things I really missed about going grain-free was a cold bowl of cereal. This recipe satisfied my craving and is so easy to keep on hand in the refrigerator.

It has all of the elements of a great cereal and packs a nutrient filled punch to your morning. You can also pack this up for a great snack during the day, or if out hiking or adventuring.

Prep time: 2 mins   *Serves: 1-2*

Directions:

Measure the nuts into a bowl and soak at least 20 minutes. You can soak overnight for greater taste and when soaked, nuts and seeds will begin the sprouting process which bumps up their nutrient profile considerably.

Preheat oven to 325°F. Line a baking sheet with parchment paper.

Drain the nuts and place in food processor. Add coconut oil, honey, cinnamon, chai seeds and salt. Pulse for half a minute, until the mixture takes on a granola like consistency.

Spread the mixture evenly on the parchment paper pan. Bake 15 minutes, mix the nuts and bake for another 15 minutes. Continue to bake and mix in 5 minute increments until nuts golden.

Remove from the oven and let cool fully. Add the raisins, dates and shredded coconut.

Dish up in a small bowl with fresh berries and serve with organic sugar free coconut milk.

Ingredients:

- ½ cup pecans
- ½ cup walnuts
- ½ cup sunflower seeds
- ½ cup hazelnuts OR almonds
- ½ cup pumpkin seeds
- 3 tbsp honey
- 2 tbsp ground chai seeds
- 1 tsp cinnamon
- 2 tbsp coconut oil
- 1 cup unsweetened coconut flakes

Continued on next page

Store in the refrigerator to keep the dried fruit fresh.

Option:

You can switch out any of the ingredients. Feel free to add more of another or even a different fruit, like prune or unsweetened dried apricots or mango. I always love adding in extra dates. You can try Almonds, sliced almonds or cashews in place of any nut in this recipe. Find what works for you and dig in.

Ingredients:

➢ 1 cup raisins or mixed berries (unsweetened)

➢ 1 cup chopped Mejool dates

➢ Pink Himalayan salt to taste

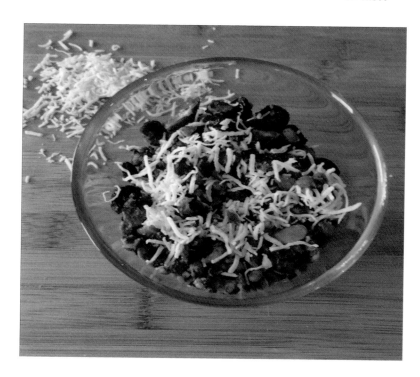

Pancakes: Banana or Sweet Potato

Who doesn't miss pancakes after going gluten and grain-free? These pancakes can be pre-made and frozen. Just pop one in the toaster oven in the morning before work or school. Simple!

So don't buy the processed frozen ones at the grocery store. Just double up on the Saturday morning pancakes and you have an easy option during the week.

Prep time: 10-15 mins   *Serves: 4-6*

Directions:

Mash bananas with fork or use 1 cup of canned organic sweet potato and put into bowl.

Beat in eggs and add the rest of the ingredients to mashed mix (If batter is too thick, add water by 1 tbsp amounts until desired thickness).

Heat olive or coconut oil in a flat pan. Pour batter onto pan in desired pancake size. Cook each side for 1-2 minutes, until slightly browned.

Serve with maple syrup and fruit.

Note:

Protein powder is available in most organic or health food stores. Look for a brand that is soy-free, dairy-free, gluten-free and make sure to avoid ingredients like rice starch/flour or corn starch as these are considered grains. If you'd rather not use protein powder, you can use coconut flour instead.

Ingredients:

➢ 4 bananas OR 1 cup of mashed canned sweet potato
➢ 6 eggs
➢ ¾ cup vanilla protein powder (or use coconut flour and 1 tsp vanilla)
➢ 1 tsp cinnamon
➢ ½ cup blueberries or chocolate chips (check for wheat or fillers)

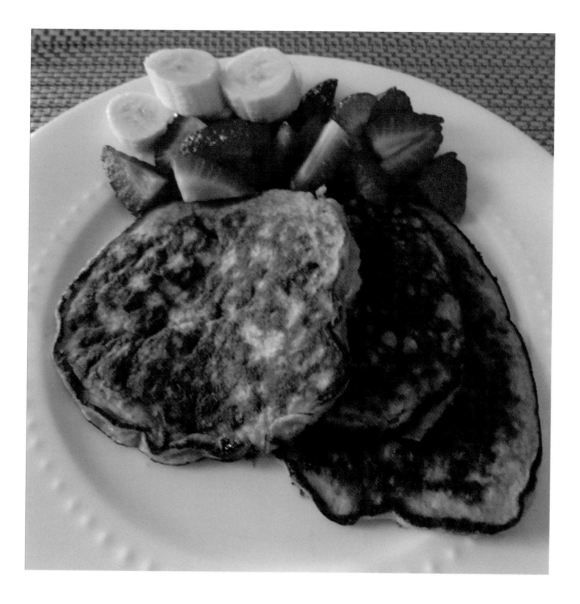

Quiche

Who says you can't enjoy quiche without flour? It's a wonderfully light egg dish that can be prepped the night before and quickly put in the oven in the morning.

This is also a great dish to whip up for lunch or dinner with a salad or some fruit.

Prep time: 10 mins   *Serves: 4-6*

Directions:

Preheat oven to 375°F

Generously grease pie pan with coconut oil.

Whisk together top ingredients and set aside.

Combine bottom ingredients and spoon into bottom of pie pan.

Pour top ingredients over bottom ingredients.

Bake 30-35 minutes until center is set. Let stand 5 minutes before serving.

Option:

Can add in ½ cup of your favorite cheese if you can handle dairy.

This recipe can be doubled easily. Just bake a little longer - 45-50 minutes.

Ingredients:

Top:
- 3 eggs
- ½ cup organic, unsweetened coconut milk
- ¼ tsp salt
- ¼ tsp pepper

Bottom:
- ½ cup cooked nitrate-free ham or bacon
- 1/3 cup chopped broccoli
- 1 spring onion

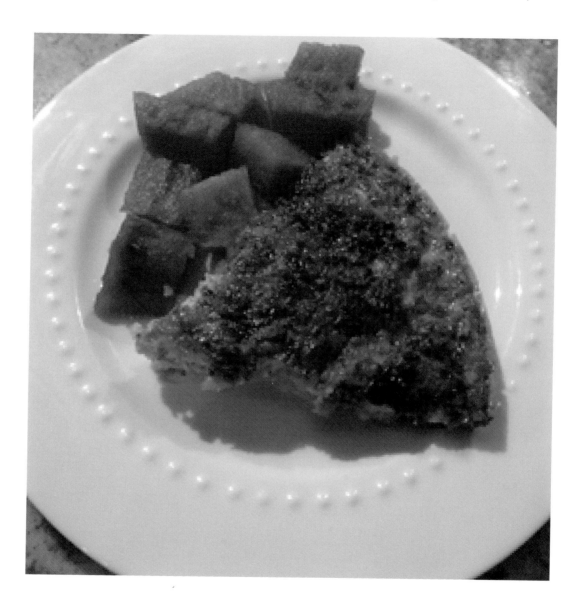

Salsa

This is a great side dish to eggs, or smoked salmon, or just on it's own.

Mix it up with different peppers and feel the difference eating fresh, raw produce can make for your body first thing in the morning.

Prep time: 10 mins   *Serves: 3-4*

Directions:

Slice up peppers, cucumber and onion and place in bowl.

Crush garlic and add to veggie mixture.

Add tomato and Himalayan Pink Crystal salt.

Drizzle lemon juice last and toss and serve.

Option:

Can substitute any of the peppers for others to your liking. I like having a lot of color so mixed it up, but you could use a whole red, yellow or orange pepper instead.

Note:

White table salt is devoid of the full spectrum of minerals and other nutrients that protect and enhance your health.
Himalayan Pink Crystal salt it contains the full spectrum of 84 minerals and trace elements just like Mother Earth intended.

Ingredients:

- ½ yellow pepper
- ½ orange pepper
- ½ hot pepper of your choice (optional)
- 1 mini cucumber
- 1 small onion
- 3-4 cloves garlic
- 2-3 tbsp lemon juice
- 1 cup roma tomatoes
- Himalayan Pink Crystal salt to taste

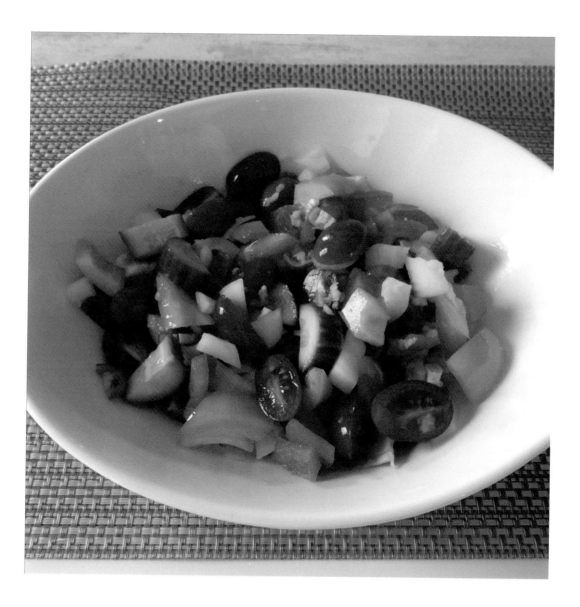

Smoked Salmon

Smoked salmon is a "superfood" with multiple health benefits, such as a great source of protein, the antioxidant vitamin E, vitamin B-12 and omega-3 fatty acids.

This is an awesome breakfast and I like to have with a big serving of fresh salsa from the previous recipe in this cook book.

Prep time: 3 mins   *Serves: 1-2*

Directions:

Open smoked salmon and place on plate.

Chop red onion and sprinkle over smoked salmon, along with capers.

Add tomato and Himalayan Pink Crystal salt.

Drizzle lemon juice last and enjoy.

Option:

Can use other onions to your liking or omit if too strong.

Ingredients:

➢ Smoked Salmon
➢ 2 tbsp chopped red onion
➢ 1 tbsp capers
➢ ½ fresh squeezed lemon

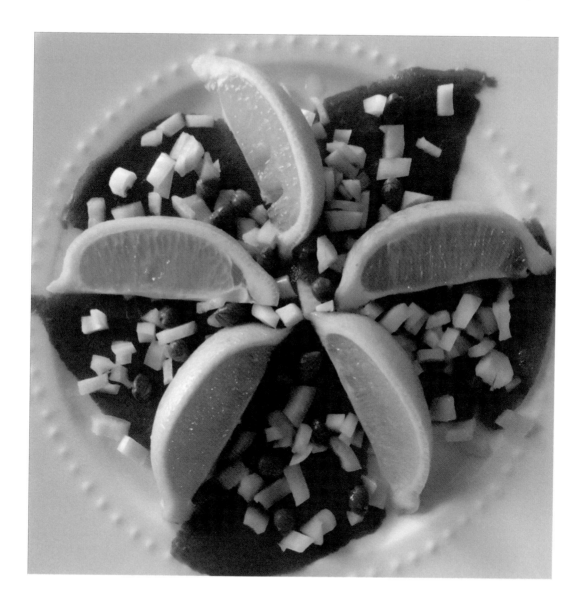

Smoothies

I struggled with how to present this recipe, as there are so many options and variations on smoothies. What it comes down to is personal liking. So I've included some guidelines here to help you establish what might work for you and your family.

Smoothies are one of the best breakfasts you can have as they maintain their nutrients from raw fruits, veggies and nuts. So mix one up and take with you if on the go.

Prep time: 5 mins   *Serves: 3-4*

Directions and guidelines:

Have a sturdy blender as part of your must haves in the kitchen.

The basics I like to always include are a handful of mixed greens, 1 banana, ½ cup mango and 1 cup of fresh or frozen berries. Place in the blender.

Add 1 cup unsweetened coconut milk.

Pour coconut water/filtered water into the blender to cover the mixture.

Add 1-2 scoops of protein powder or ¼ cup of your favorite nuts for protein. If using nuts, this will give your smoothie a bit more of a chewy texture.

My kids like a bit of sweetness to their smoothies so I then add 1-2 tbsps of honey.

Blend fully and serve in a glass, in a to go mug, or with a straw for fun.

Ingredients:

➢ Handful of mixed greens
➢ 1 banana
➢ ½ cup frozen or fresh mango
➢ 1 cup berries of your choice (blueberry, blackberry, raspberry)
➢ 1 cup unsweetened coconut milk
➢ Coconut water or filtered water

Continued on next page

Options:

Throw in a carrot and/or 1-2 tbsp fresh ginger for some extra zip.

Can also squeeze some fresh lime or lemon. Experiment and enjoy the wealth of opportunities to make smoothies a part of your morning.

Note:

Protein powder is available in most organic or health food stores. Look for a brand that is soy-free, dairy-free, gluten-free and make sure to avoid ingredients like rice starch/flour or corn starch as these are considered grains.

Ingredients:

➢ 1-2 scoops protein powder or nuts

➢ 1-2 tbsp honey to taste (optional)

Caution:

The dark side of kale and spinach - it's important to understand what kale - and the whole family of cruciferous vegetables - might be doing to your thyroid, and how to safely incorporate these powerhouse foods into your diet. I have a thyroid issue so avoid a lot of spinach and kale in my smoothies. But do your own research, consult with your health care professional and be informed.

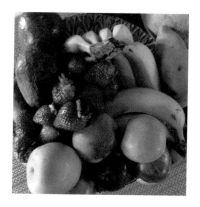

Source - http://thyroid.about.com/b/2014/01/14/the-dark-side-of-kale-spinach-broccoli-etc-thyroid-disease.htm

Sweet Potato Hash Scramble

This is so delicious and a great way to use up left-over sweet potato or potatoes.

I also like to sprinkle turmeric on many of my vegetables as it's known to help enhance the body's immune system. So sprinkle away and enjoy breakfast!

Prep time: 10 mins   *Serves: 1-2*

Directions:

Peel and cut sweet potato into 1" cubes.

Put 1-2 tbsp olive oil in pan. Place the potato, chopped spring onion, salt and pepper and turmeric in the pan.

On medium heat, cover and cook until potato is soft, stirring occasionally (Approximately 10-15 mins). You can add a bit of butter if you like.

Remove lid, and move potato mixture around in the pan to make 2 holes.

Crack the eggs into the holes and cover pan until eggs are cooked to desired consistency.

Option:

You can use up any left over baked or boiled potatoes you have in the fridge. Slice them in bite-sized pieces and your cooking time will be reduced as they are already cooked.

Ingredients:

➢ 1 medium sweet potato
➢ 1-2 tbsp olive oil
➢ 2 eggs
➢ 1 spring onion
➢ Salt and pepper to taste
➢ 1 tsp turmeric

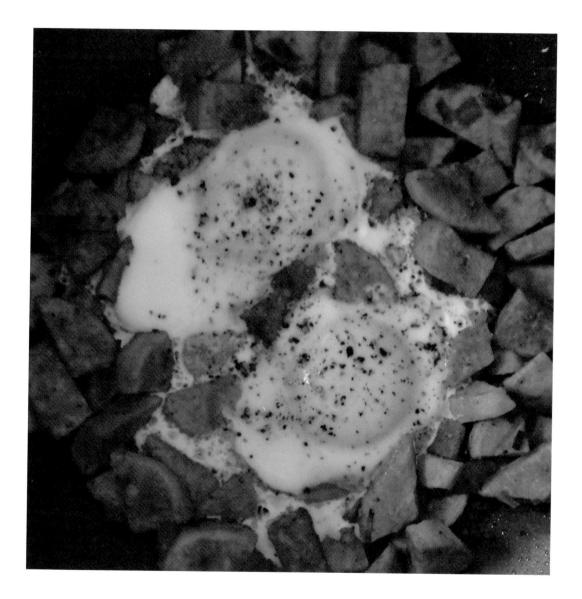

Tea; Ginger, Lemon and Honey

Among the many health benefits of honey, what is most impressive to me is that honey can be a powerful immune system booster. It's antioxidant and anti-bacterial properties can help improve the digestive system and help you stay healthy and fight disease.

And how about Ginger? Well, I think the most impressive benefit is it is ideal in assisting digestion, thereby improving food absorption and avoiding possible stomach ache.

So start your day with this lovely tea and reap the health benefits from drinking it.

Prep time: 5 mins   *Serves: 1*

Directions:

Put your kettle on to boil water.

Peel and cut ginger into small pieces and place in a tea cup.

Measure out 1-2 tsp of honey, depending on how sweet you want it. Place in the tea cup with the ginger and add your freshly squeezed lemon.

Pour boiling water in the cup when ready, and let steep for 5 minutes.

Note:

You can put the ginger in a sieve and remove after steeping your tea, or leave in and eat. I enjoy the tanginess and little bit of zip that ginger gives so prefer to eat, but it can be strong for some.

Ingredients:

➤ 1-2 tbsp ginger
➤ 1-2 tsp honey
➤ ½ fresh lemon
➤ Boiling water

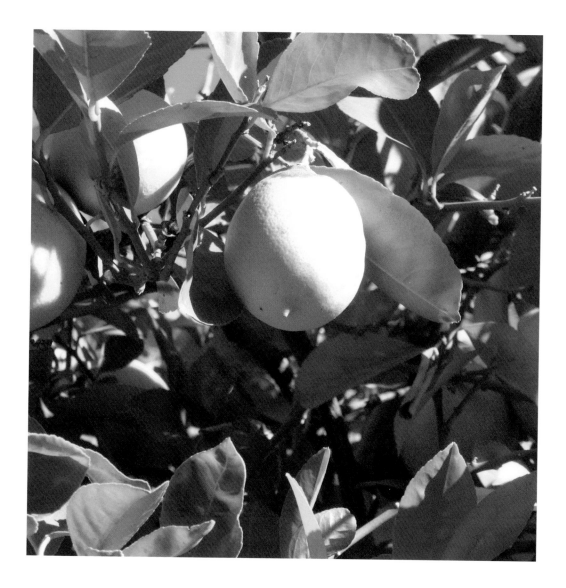

Final Note

Remember you are not alone on this journey. There will be many people who view the way you eat as "not healthy" or "weird". But know that as you take this journey to regain your health, you are doing what is right for you and your body, mind and spirit. Appreciate the concerns of others, but ultimately know that you are not alone. Most of the people in my life are not gluten-free or celiac, and really do not understand. But if those in your life care about you they will be supportive.

I wanted to share a final story with you. Recently I got a stomach bug (my son had it the week before and it had been going around our school). I haven't gotten this sick in a number of years. My best and most supportive friend in so many ways was very worried about me. She said maybe I should get off this "health kick" and start eating normal again. I know she loves me and is just concerned about me, but like so many others has a hard time understanding.

It is at times like this that I feel very alone. But I also look at it as an opportunity to share with others that we are all unique and different. I eat gluten and grain-free not as a lifestyle choice, but out of necessity. And the reality is even if you don't react to grains, you probably are getting more grains in your diet than you need. Fruits and vegetables are the key. The Canadian Food Guide recommends 7-10 servings of fruits and vegetables for adults every day. Are you getting enough? Even for those in your life who are not gluten intolerant or celiac, encourage them to look to more fresh alternatives.

I did end up going the doctor as a result of getting sick, who told me to eat BRAT (Bananas, Rice, Apples, Toast). This is what doctors are trained to tell us. When I reminded my doctor that I don't eat grains, she said to eat lots of bananas and liquids. Doctors do the best they can given their training, but I would suggest visiting a nutritionist and/or naturopath if you want a full plan for your health recovery and maintenance.

I am not a doctor, or nutritionist. The recommendations in this book are made from the sources listed in the reference section and what I have discovered on my journey with my family. If you really are struggling, please find a team of professionals you trust including holistic nutritionists, naturopaths and your family doctor.

On a final note, no one is perfect. I have healed the inflammation in my intestines and feel very healthy and good…most of the time. On occasion I do indulge in some rice-based products or the odd "gluten-free" pizza. While I find I don't react too badly with cramping, it does make me feel extremely tired and grouchy…almost like a hangover. So if you do indulge don't feel guilty, but do know the ramifications of the end result from that treat.

All the best to you as you reclaim energy and health with the most important meal of the day!

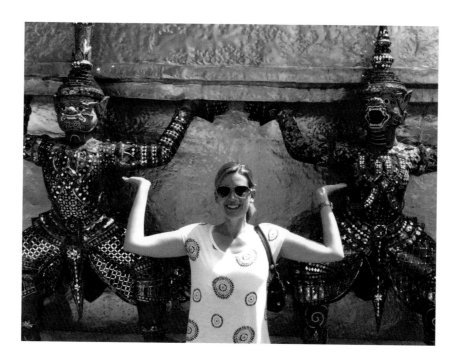

Conversions

VOLUMES

US	METRIC
1 tsp	5 ml
1 tbsp ((1/2 fl ox)	15 ml
¼ cup (2 fl oz)	60 ml
1/3 cup	80 ml
½ cup (4 fl oz)	120 ml
2/3 cup	160ml
¾ cup (6 fl oz)	180 ml
1 cup (8 fl oz)	240 ml
1 qt + 3 tbsps	1 L
1 gal (128 fl oz)	4 L

TEMPERATURES

Fahrenheit	Celsius
0°	-18°
32°	0°
180°	82°
212°	100°
250°	120°
350°	175°
425°	220°
500°	260°

WEIGHTS

US	METRIC
¼ oz	7 g
½ oz	15 g
¾ oz	20 g
1 oz	30 g
8 oz (1/2 lb)	225 g
12 oz (3/4 lb)	340 g
16 oz (1 lb)	455 g
35 oz (2.2 lbs)	1 kg

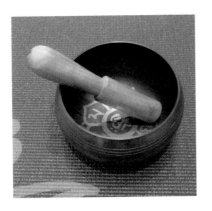

References

Here are some references that I thought you might find useful. This list is far from exhaustive, with new sites and information being launched constantly. But these are a few that I thought you might like to start investigating.

Informational Websites

www.glutenfreesociety.org - Resource on all things gluten! Video tutorials, Interactive Forum, Gluten Intolerance Testing, and more.

http://www.celiac.com/ - A invaluable resource to people worldwide who seek information about celiac disease and related disorders.

https://gfafexpo.com/ - The Expo is the premier gluten and allergen free event in the US.

http://www.glutenfreeexpo.ca/ - Expanded across Canada to connect with more members of the Gluten Free community.

http://www.articlesofhealth.blogspot.ca/ - The writings of Robert O. Young D.Sc., Ph.D., based upon his theory that the human organism is alkaline by design and acidic by function.

Recipe and Product Websites:

http://detoxinista.com/special-diets/paleo-friendly/ - Recipes are all gluten-free and refined sugar-free, and many of them are also raw, vegan, and Paleo-friendly.

http://www.thepaleomom.com/ - A scientist turned stay-at-home mom who shares recipes, explains the science behind the paleo diet and its modifications, and blogs about the challenges of raising a paleo family.

www.iherb.com - A robust selection of natural products and vitamins and they will ship internationally within a few days.

http://www.miraclenoodle.com/default.aspx - The fiber found in Miracle Noodle slows digestion and prolongs the sensation of fullness. Can also be ordered on iherb.com.

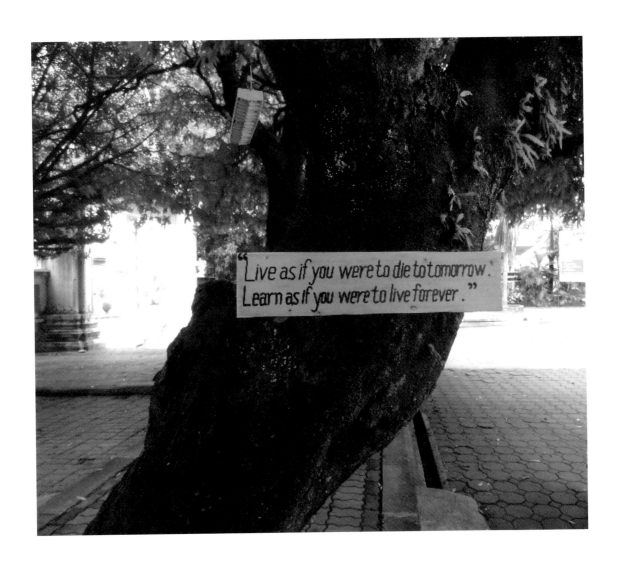

Glossary

The source of definitions below has been taken from the on-line resource Wikipedia. Please refer to this site for full detailed definitions and references.

Acidic - a chemical substance characterized by a sour taste, the ability to turn blue litmus red, and the ability to react with bases and certain metals (like calcium) to form salts. Aqueous solutions of acids have a pH of less than 7. A lower pH means a higher acidity, and thus a higher concentration of positive hydrogen ions in the solution. Chemicals or substances having the property of an acid are said to be acidic.

Allergy - a hypersensitivity disorder of the immune system. Symptoms include red eyes, itchiness, and runny nose, eczema, hives, or an asthma attack.

Alkalinity - Measures the ability of a solution to neutralize acids to the equivalence point of carbonate or bicarbonate.

Antibacterial - a type of antimicrobial used specifically against bacteria, and are often used in medical treatment of bacterial infections. They may either kill or inhibit the growth of bacteria.

Antioxidant - a molecule that inhibits the oxidation of other molecules.

Bacteria - microorganisms. Typically a few micrometers in length, bacteria have a number of shapes, ranging from spheres to rods and spirals. Bacteria were among the first life forms to appear on Earth, and are present in most of its habitats. Bacteria inhabit soil, water, acidic hot springs, radioactive waste, and the deep portions of Earth's crust. Bacteria also live in symbiotic and parasitic relationships with plants and animals.

Celiac Disease - an autoimmune disorder of the small intestine that occurs in genetically predisposed people of all ages from middle infancy onward. Symptoms include pain and discomfort in the digestive tract, chronic constipation and diarrhea, failure to thrive (in children), anemia and fatigue, but these may be absent, and symptoms in other organ systems have been described. Vitamin deficiencies are often noted in people with celiac disease owing to the reduced ability of the small intestine to properly absorb nutrients from food.

Gluten - a protein composite found in wheat and related grains, including barley and rye. Gluten is the composite of a gliadin and a glutenin, which is conjoined with starch in the endosperm of various grass-related grains.

Gluten-Free - A gluten-free diet is a diet that excludes gluten, a protein composite found in wheat and related grains, including barley and rye. Gluten causes health problems in sufferers of celiac disease (CD) and some cases of wheat allergy. For those diagnosed with celiac disease, a strict gluten-free diet constitutes the only effective treatment to date.

Gluten Intolerant - the umbrella term for all diseases triggered by gluten. Gluten-related disorders include celiac disease and non-celiac gluten sensitivity (NCGS). Formerly, also gluten intolerance has been used as umbrella term, and the expression gluten sensitivity has been used either as umbrella term or for NCGS. Symptoms include bloating, abdominal discomfort or pain, diarrhea, constipation, muscular disturbances, headaches, migraines, severe acne, fatigue, and bone or joint pain.

Grain - small, hard, dry seeds, with or without attached hulls or fruit layers, harvested for human or animal consumption. Agronomists also call the plants producing such seeds "grain crops". The two main types of commercial grain crops are cereals such as wheat and rye, and legumes such as beans and soybeans.

Irritable Bowel Syndrome (IBS) - a symptom-based diagnosis. It is characterized by chronic abdominal pain, discomfort, bloating, and alteration of bowel habits. Diarrhea or constipation may predominate, or they may alternate.

Lactose intolerant - inability of adults to digest lactose, a sugar found in milk and to a lesser extent dairy products, causing side effects. It is common for patients with inflammatory bowel disease to experience gastrointestinal symptoms after lactose ingestion.

Legume - Legumes are grown agriculturally, primarily for their food grain seed (e.g., beans and lentils). Legumes are notable in that most of them have symbiotic nitrogen-fixing bacteria in structures called root nodules. Well-known legumes include alfalfa, clover, peas, beans, lentils, lupins, mesquite, carob, soybeans, peanuts, tamarind, and the woody climbing vine wisteria.

Paleo - a modern nutritional diet designed to emulate, insofar as possible using modern foods, the diet of wild plants and animals eaten by humans during the Paleolithic era. Proponents of the diet therefore recommend avoiding any foods that they claim were not available to humans at that time, including dairy products, grains, legumes, processed oils, and refined sugar.

PH - In chemistry, pH is a measure of the acidity or basicity of an aqueous solution. Solutions with a pH less than 7 are said to be acidic and solutions with a pH greater than 7 are basic or alkaline. Pure water has a pH very close to 7. Too Much Acid in Your Body Can Cause a Host of Health Problems.

Prebiotic - non-digestible food ingredients.

Probiotic - Probiotics are microorganisms that are believed to provide health benefits when consumed. Commonly claimed benefits of probiotics include the decrease of potentially pathogenic gastro-intestinal microorganisms; the reduction of gastro-intestinal discomfort; the strengthening of the immune system; the improvement of the skin's function; the improvement of bowel regularity; the strengthening of the resistance to cedar pollen allergens; the decrease in body pathogens; the reduction of flatulence and bloating; the protection of DNA; the protection of proteins and lipids from oxidative damage; and the maintaining of individual intestinal microbiota in subjects receiving antibiotic treatment.

Vegan - the practice of abstaining from the use of all animal products, particularly in diet, as well as following an associated philosophy that rejects the commodity status of sentient animals. A follower of veganism is known as a vegan.

Vegetarian - the practice of abstaining from the consumption of meat (red meat, poultry, seafood and the flesh of any other animal), and may also include abstention from by-products of animal slaughter.